Endorsements
For Helpful Harry

'In this fun and educational book, learn the important role the tongue plays in helping with things you would expect, like feeding and speaking, but also with things you might be surprised about, such as breathing and jaw growth and development. I hope many families enjoy this tale of adventure.'

Dr David McIntosh
Paediatric airway ENT Specialist

'This book offers a playfulness that would reach young readers for the concepts we are all trying to teach. This book is so much fun. I love the careful consideration of the characters and how they interact. I was immediately drawn to the concept of a close friendship and connection between Polly and Harry. The way these characters paint a playful picture of the world within the mouth are thought provoking for young minds. The story presents common challenges in the growing mouth that children may recognise as factors in their own life. I love how Harry summons the strength and motivation to fix his own problem. The concept of finding strength to work and practice is a therapist's dream. Harry's work to reach his goals is captivating and engaging. Perhaps qualities we are trying to instill in young minds that reach far wider than just the mouth.'

Tess Norris
Cert OMT and IAOM Australian Association of Orofacial Myology President

For my children and husband
who instilled the drive for knowledge and nurtured my creative expression to better educate others.
A heartfelt thanks to my peers and mentors
who have supported my journey and helped breathe life into these pages.

Chantelle

Text & Illustrations copyright © 2025 Chantelle Nowicki

ISBN Hardback: 978-1-7640547-0-6
ISBN Paperback: 978-1-7640547-1-3
ISBN eBook 978-1-7640547-2-0

www.orofacialmyologyadelaide.com

Illustrations and design by Vaughan Duck
www.vaughanduck.com

The Tale of a
TONGUE

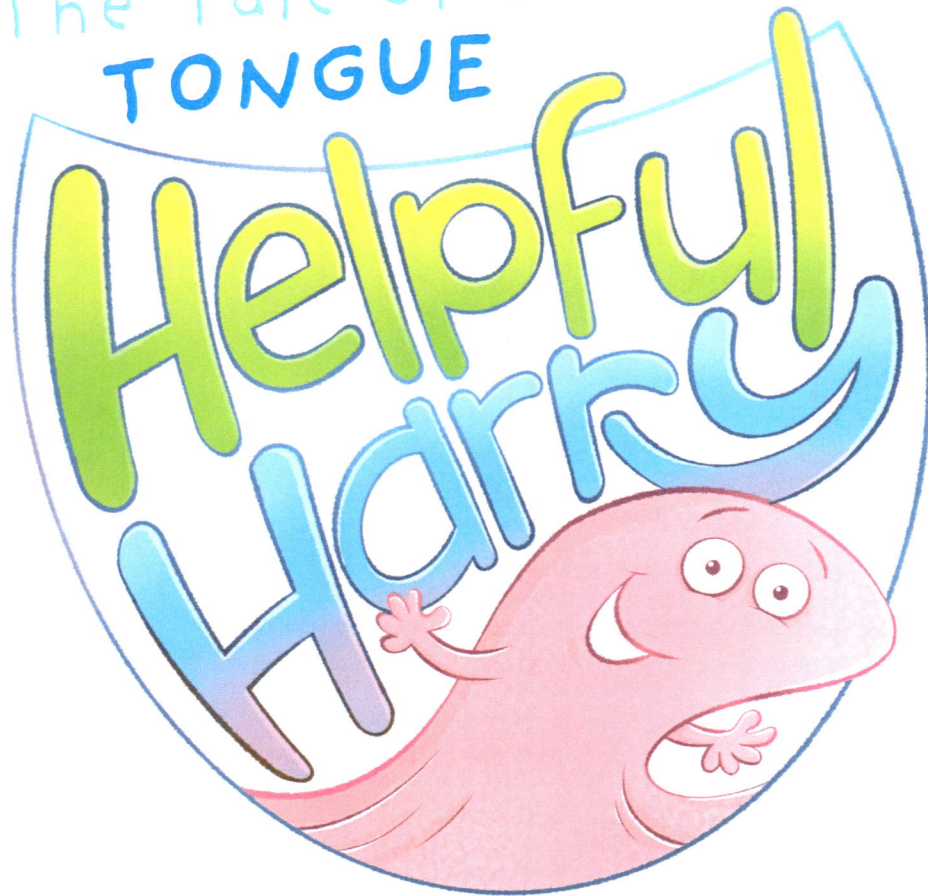

Helpful Harry

Chantelle Nowicki

illustrated by Vaughan Duck

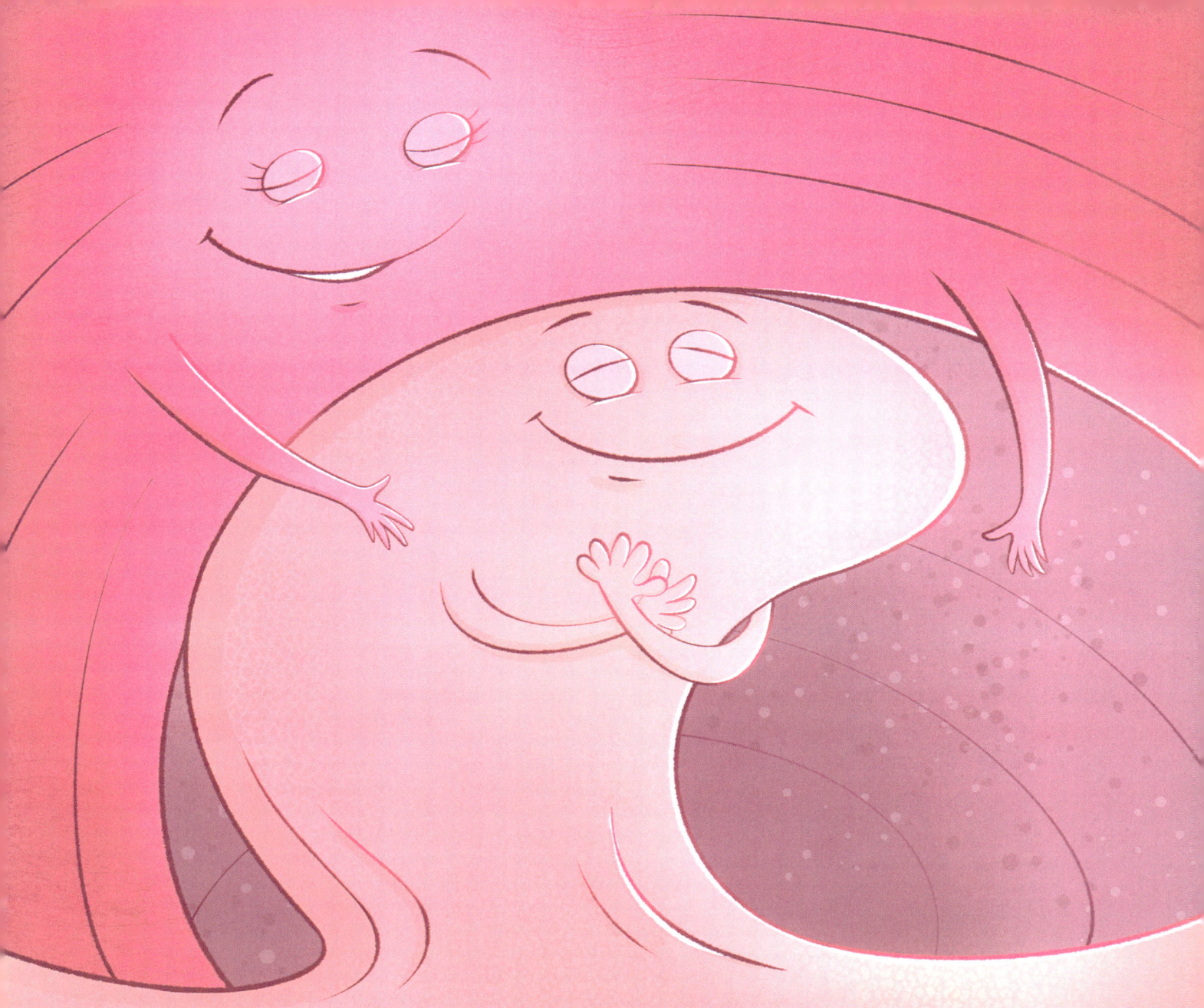

Harry and Polly, the greatest of friends,
They cuddle together, with all the right bends.

Helpful Harry,
as strong as can be.

He lifts Polly Palate
and keeps our nose free.

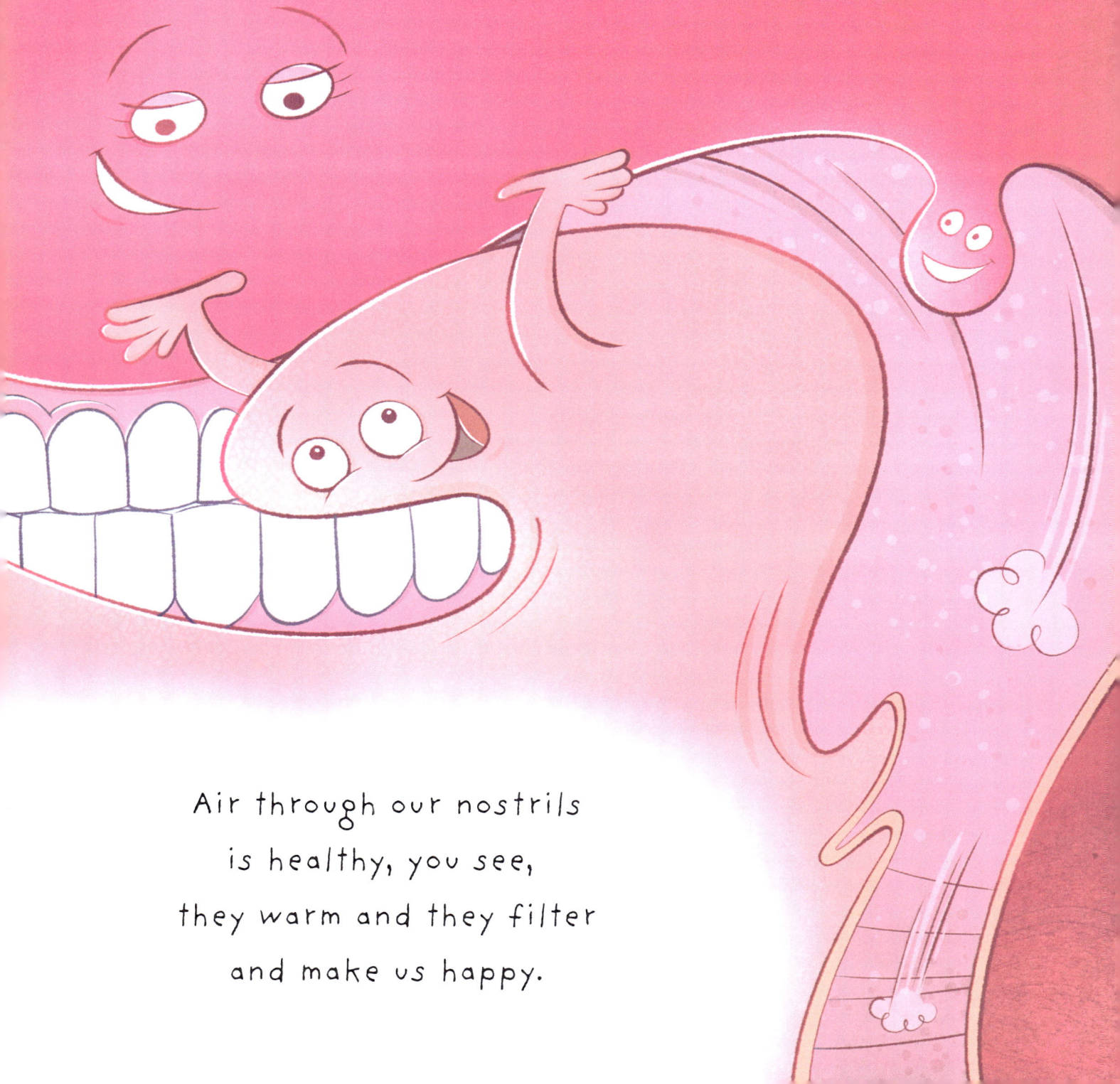

Air through our nostrils
is healthy, you see,
they warm and they filter
and make us happy.

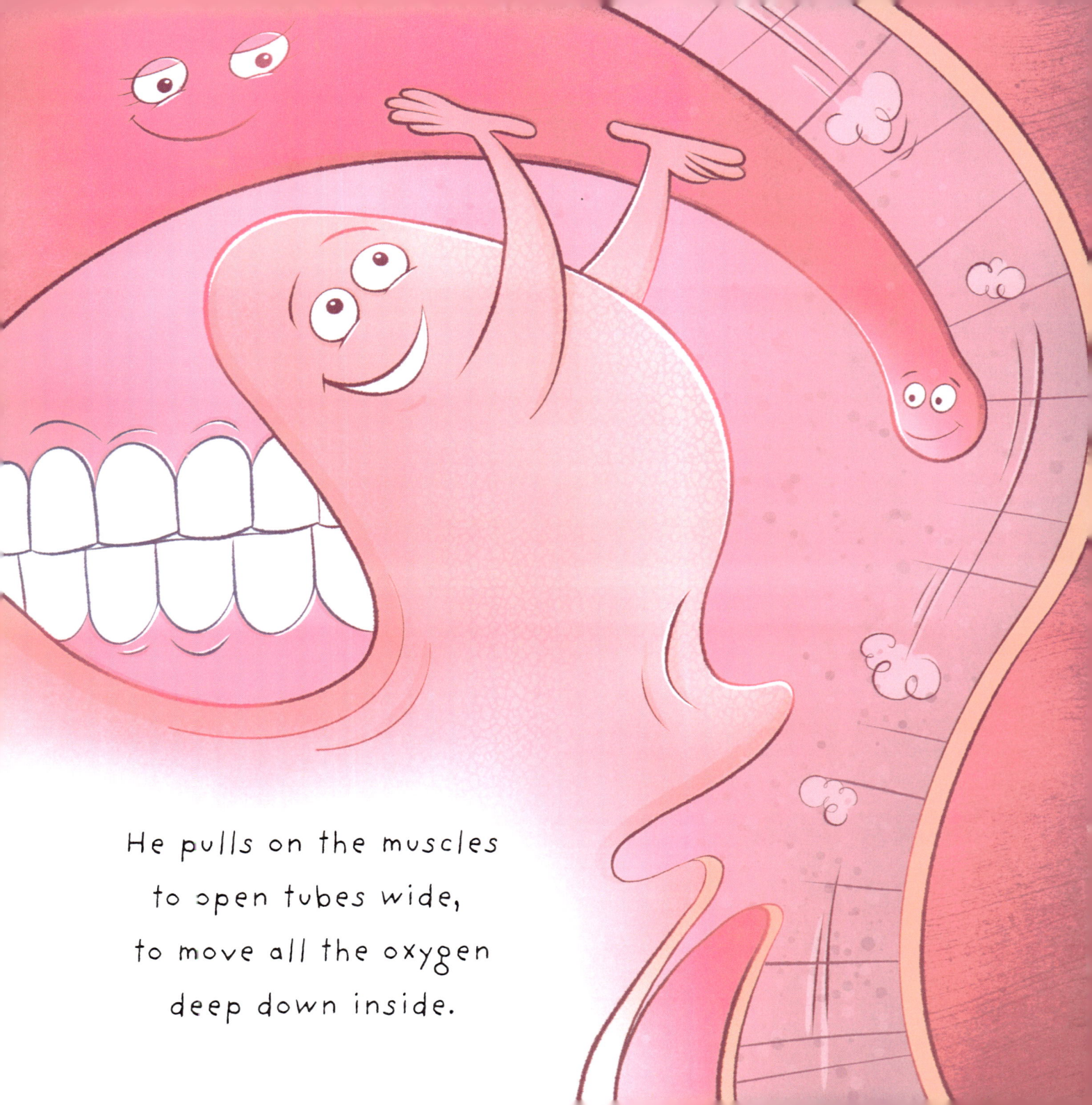

He pulls on the muscles
to open tubes wide,
to move all the oxygen
deep down inside.

He traps our food to swallow it down,

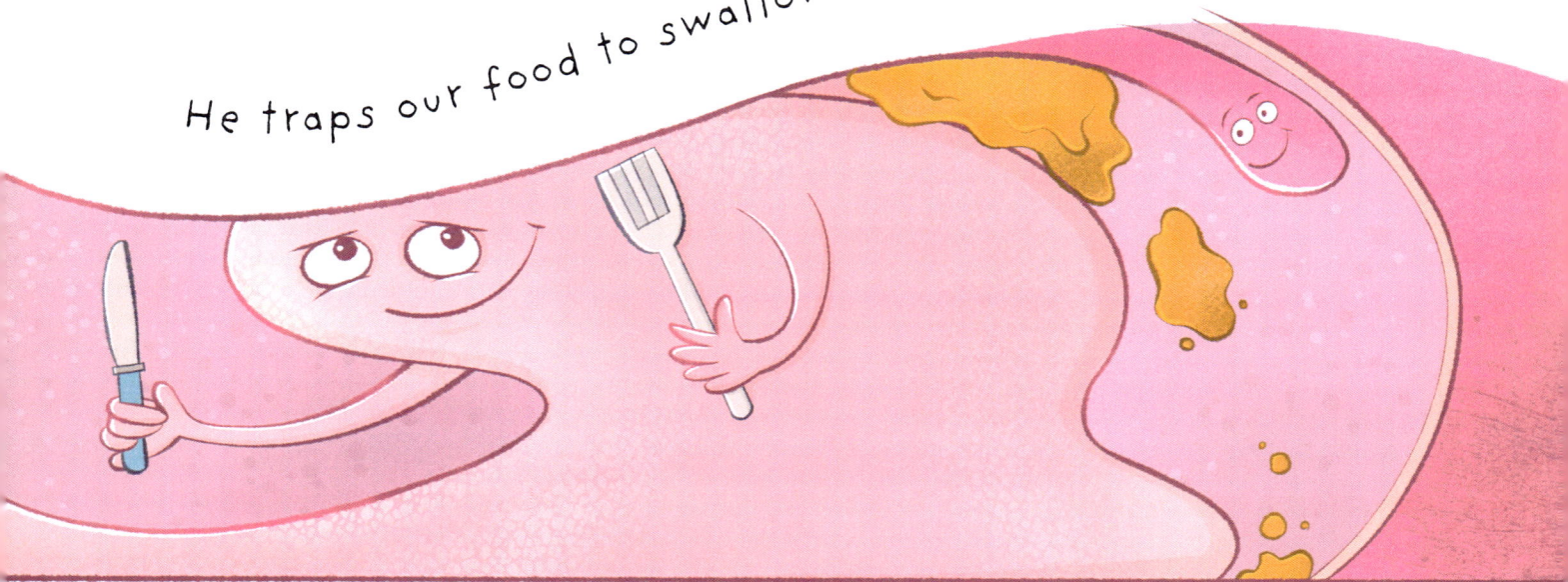

and catches our drinks, so we won't drown!

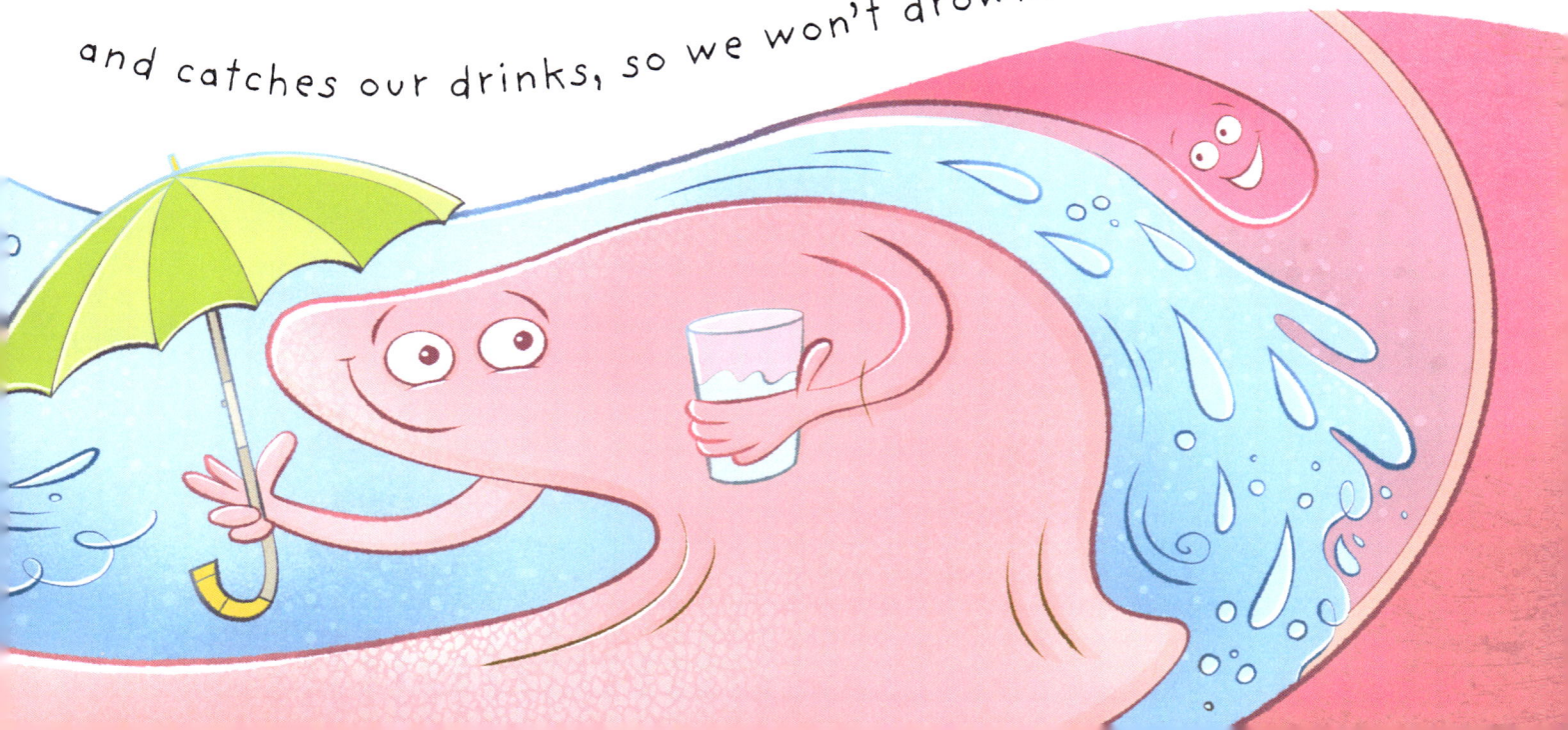

Harry's an expert
at cleaning around,
to get rid of food
and yucky things found.

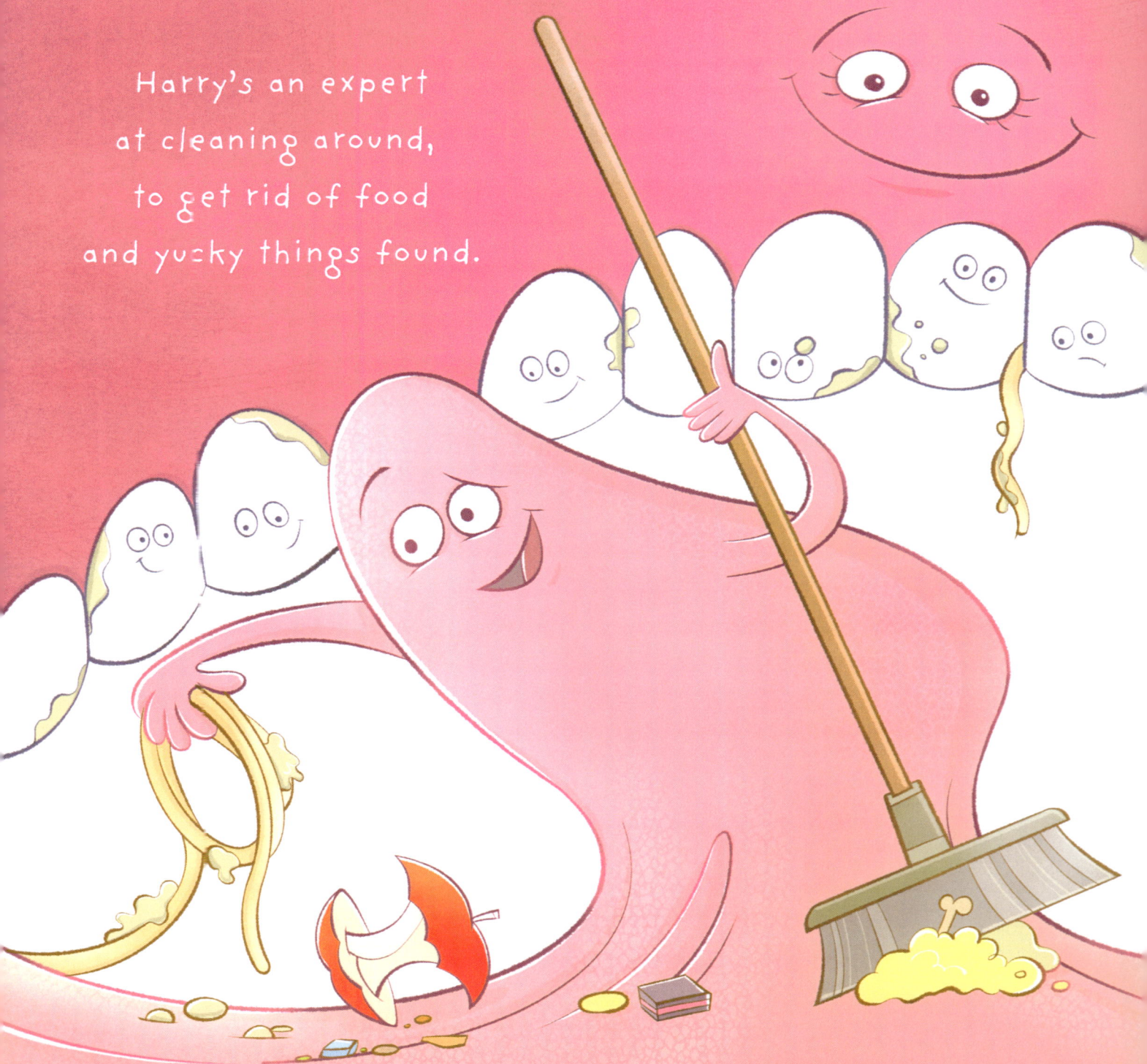

He loves a good scrub from his head to his toe,

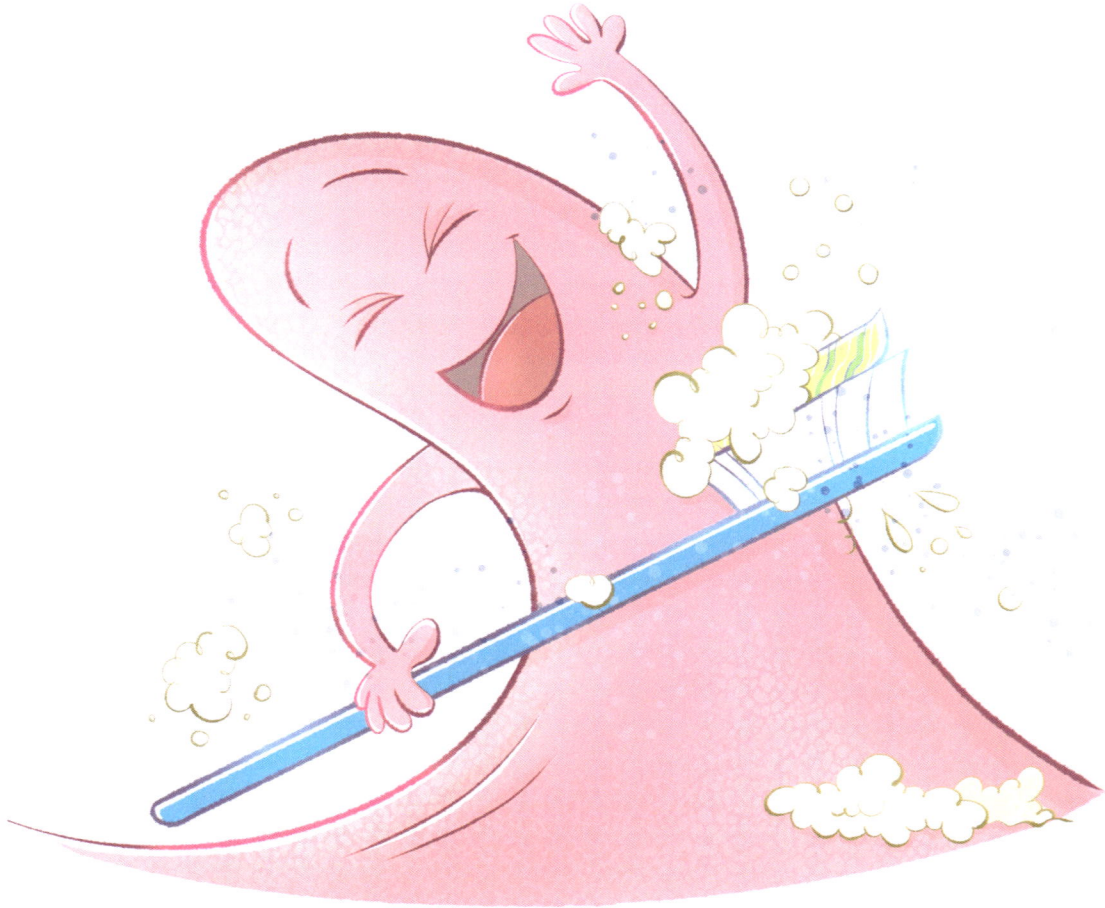

but don't clean too far cause he might just go...

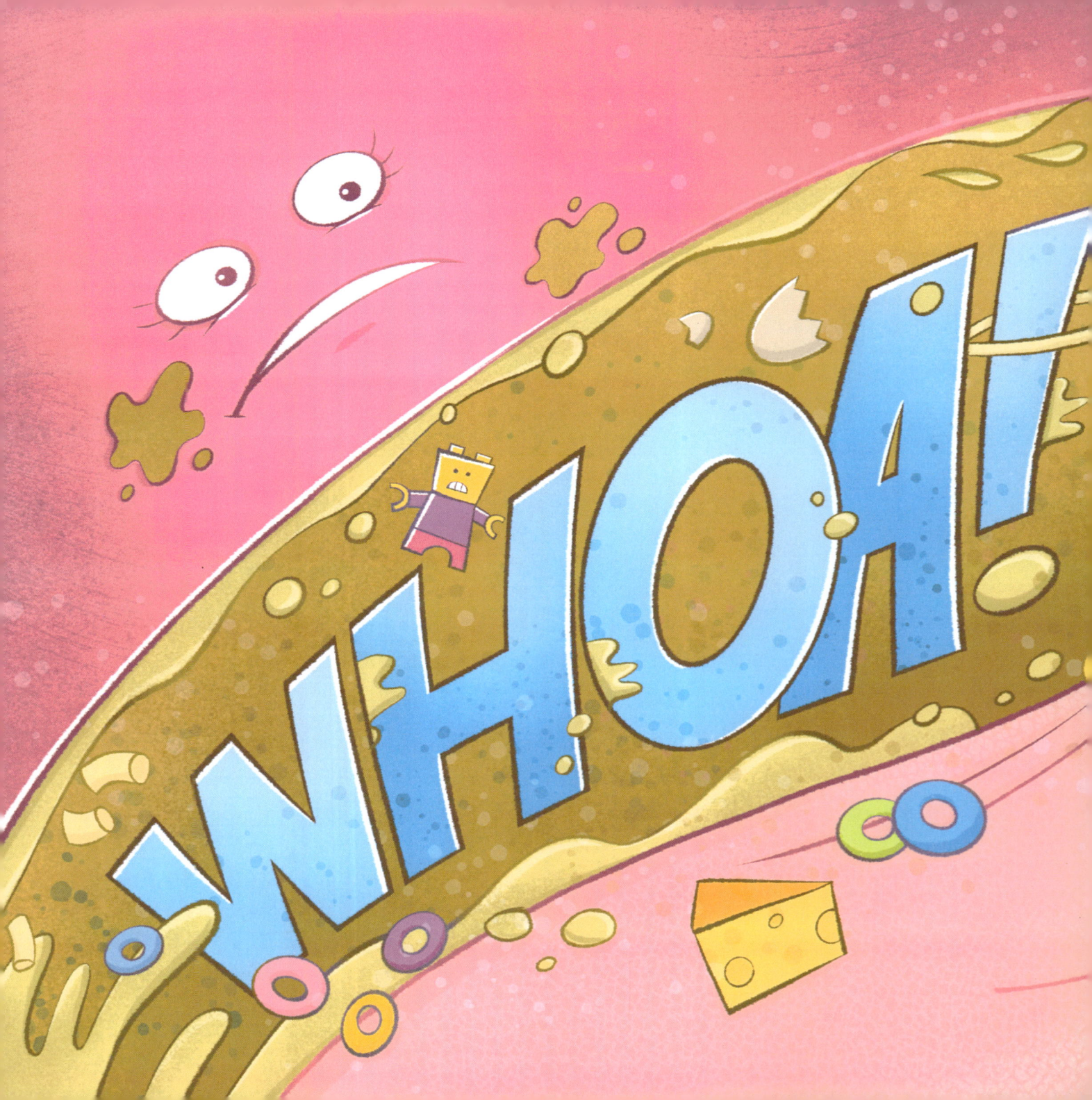

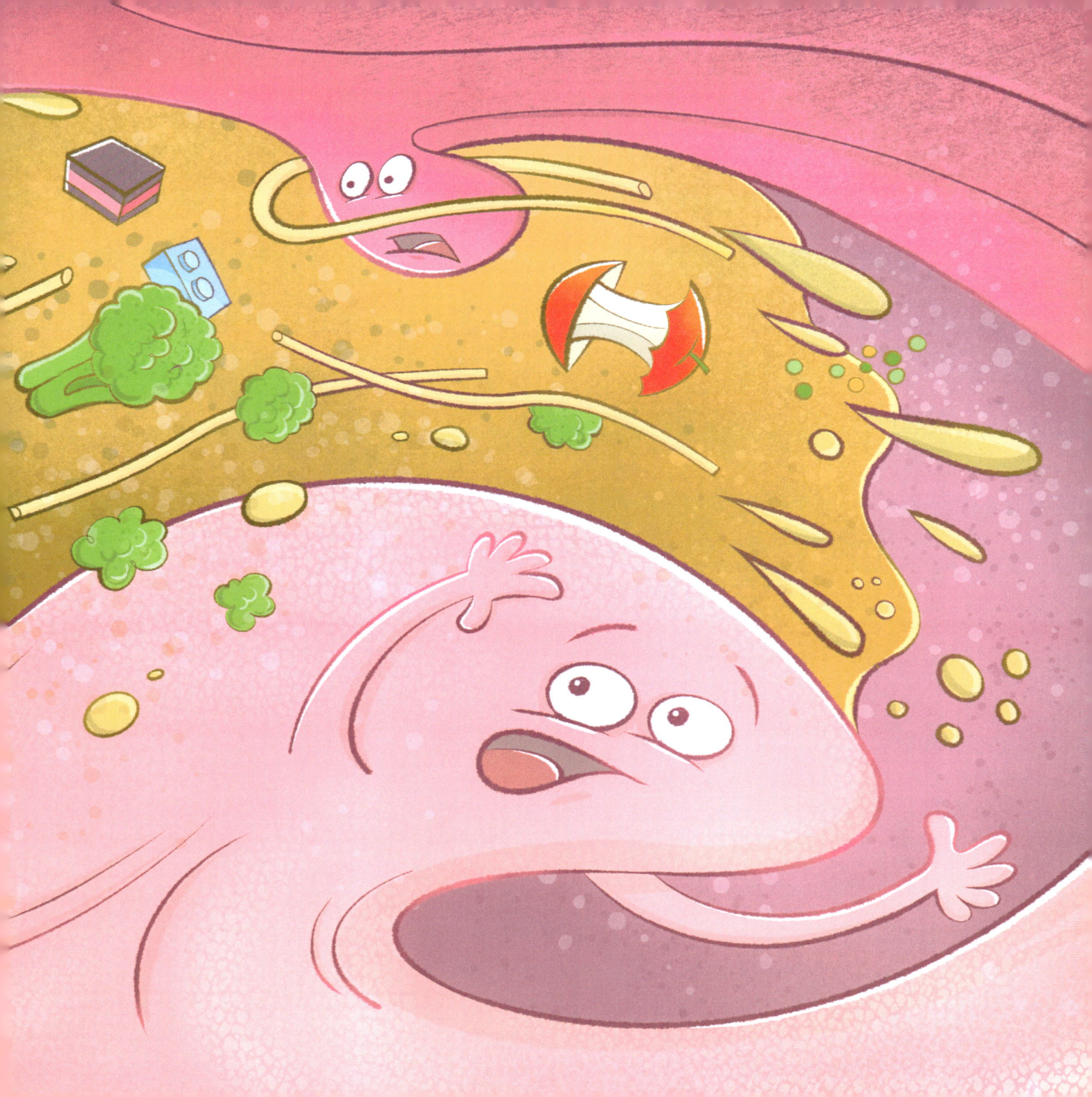

The dummies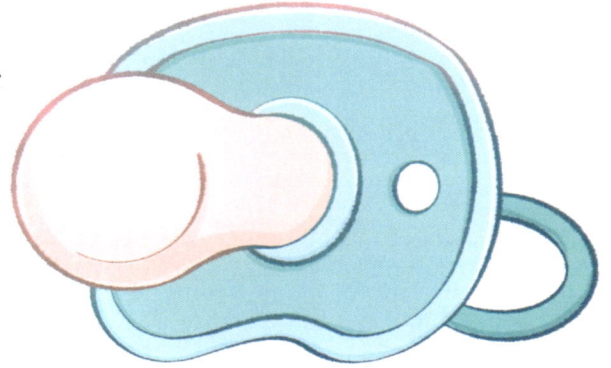

and bottles

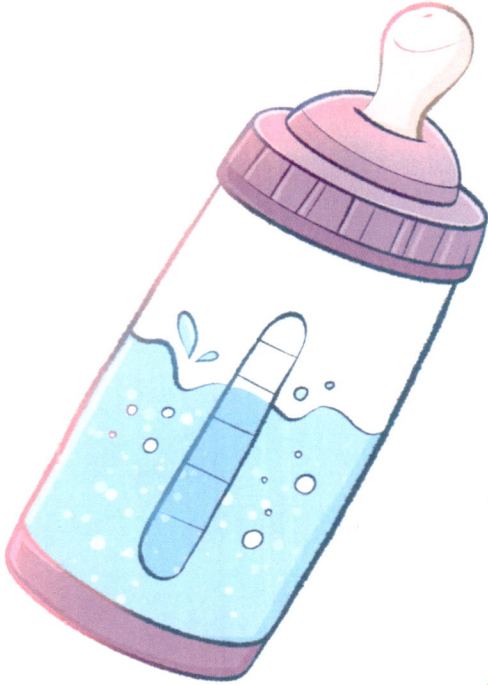

and fingers
move in,

they squish Polly Palate
and change
our nice grin.

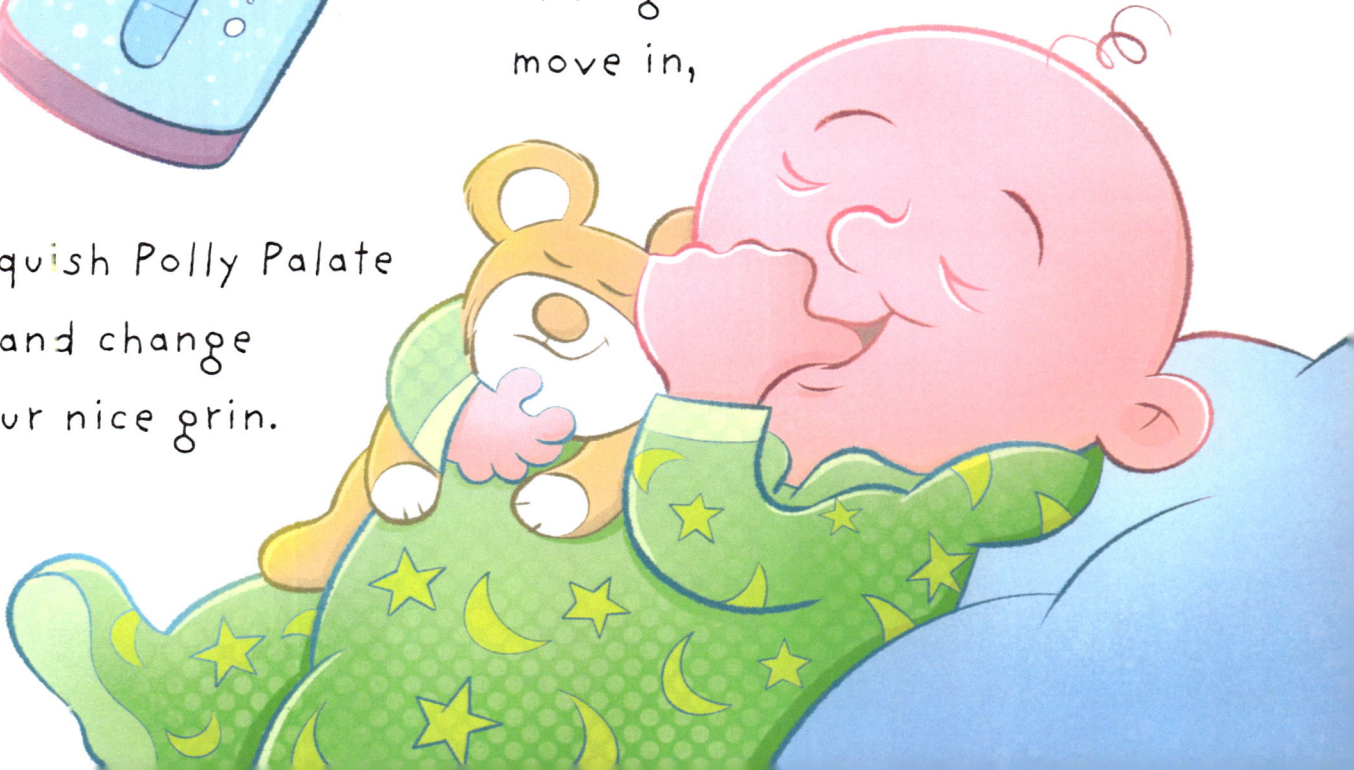

Poor Polly, so sad,
pulls away from her mate,
won't stick to dear Harry,
like old sticky tape.

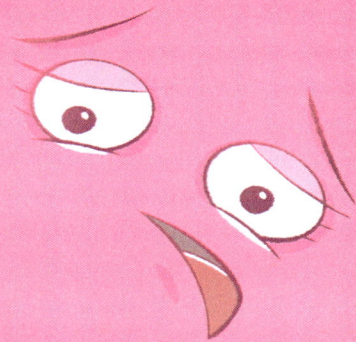

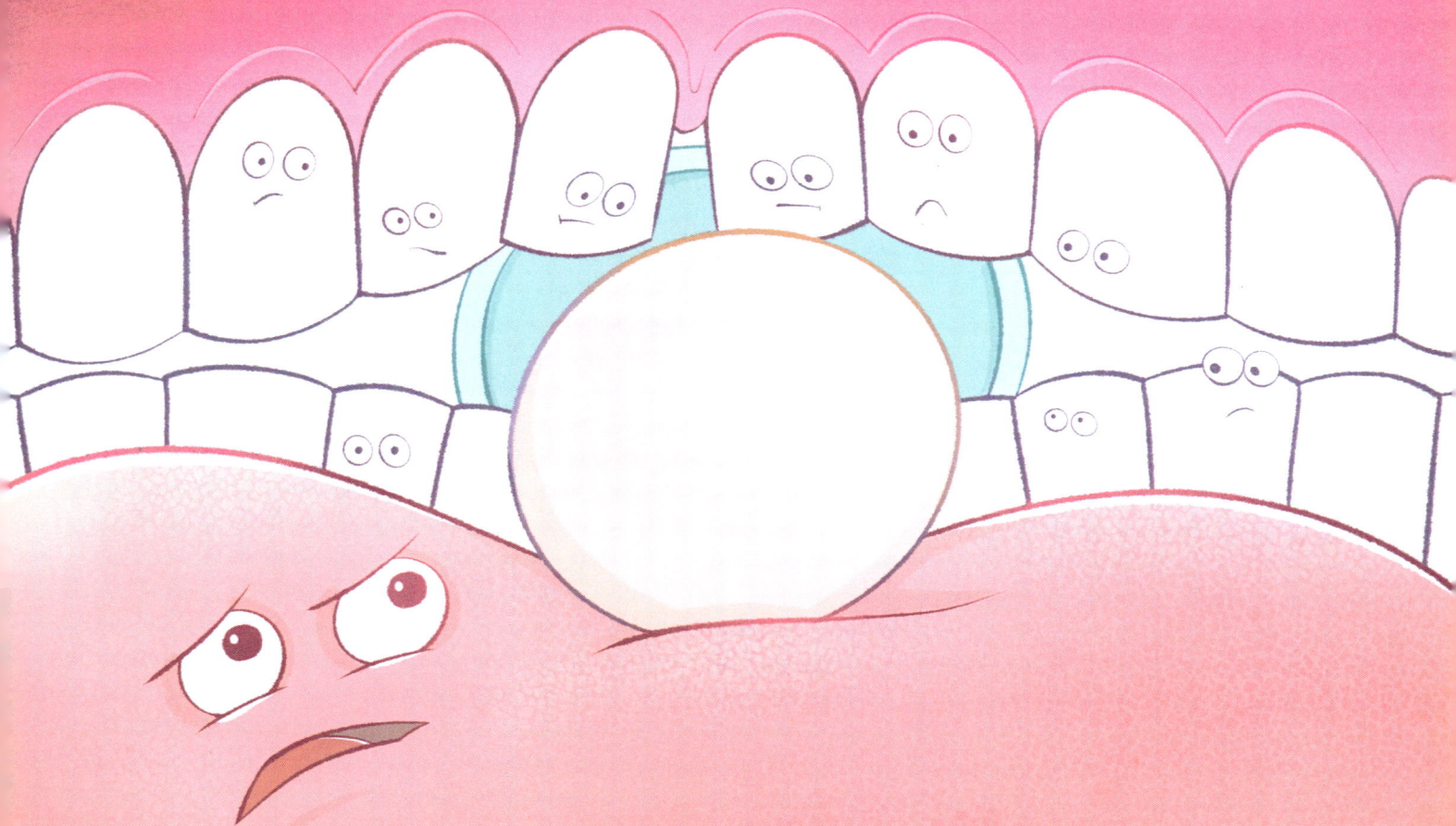

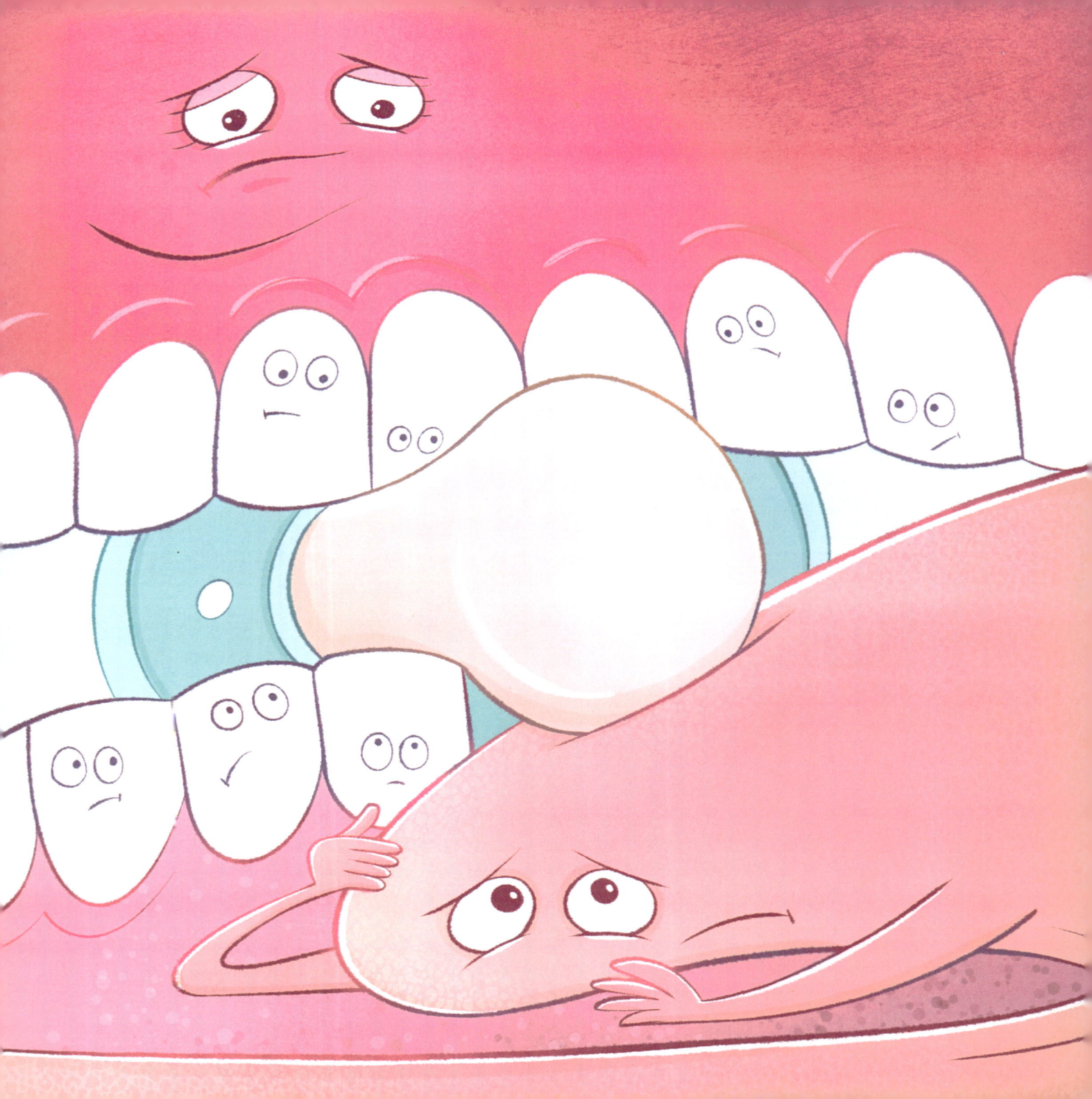

New friends arrive, with excitement and fun.
But pushing and poking leaves Harry undone.

Poor Harry, pushed far, down to the floor,
Away from Miss Polly, and opens the door...

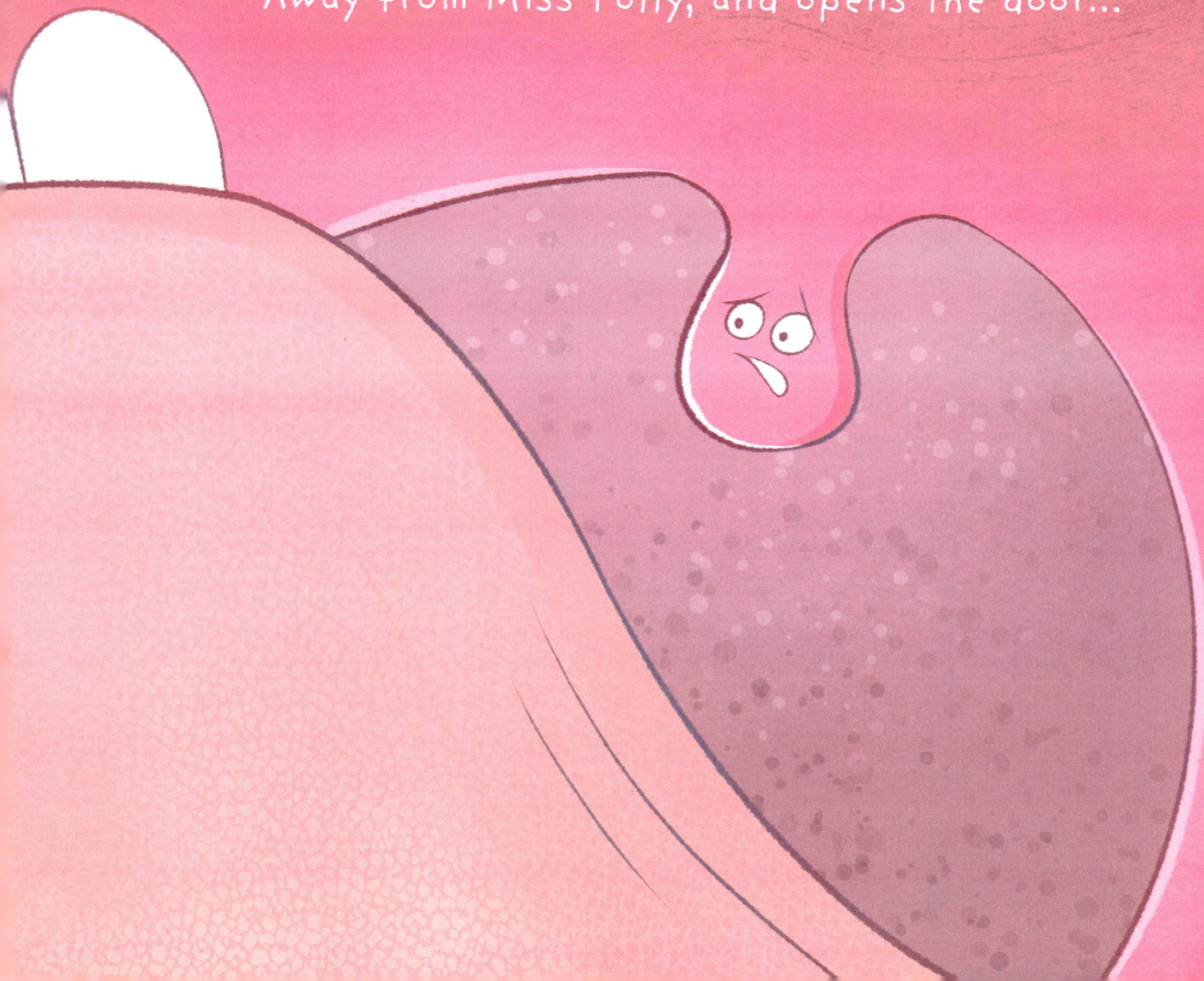

In come the nasties, from dusk until dawn.
They gather and party, jump in with a yawn.

They fill all the spaces
and pipes with a pong,

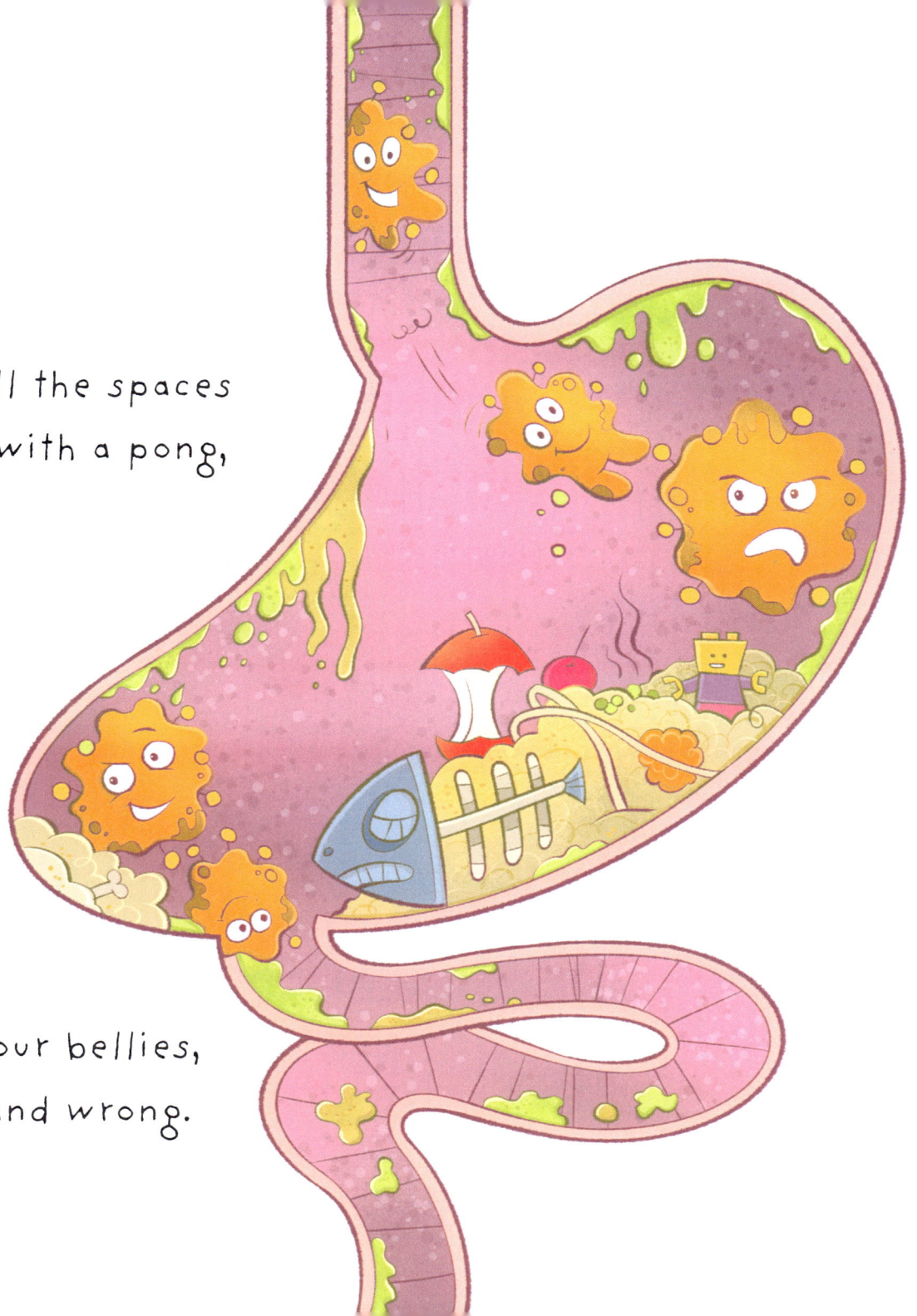

And upset our bellies,
so stinky and wrong.

Our tonsils grow larger,
the adenoids do too,
and all these new lumps
make it harder to chew!

The wind makes a whistle
deep down in our throat,
our teeth bump and chatter,
we sound like a

GOAT!

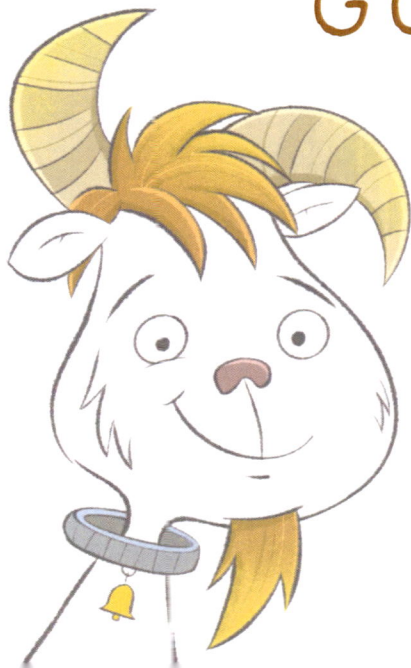

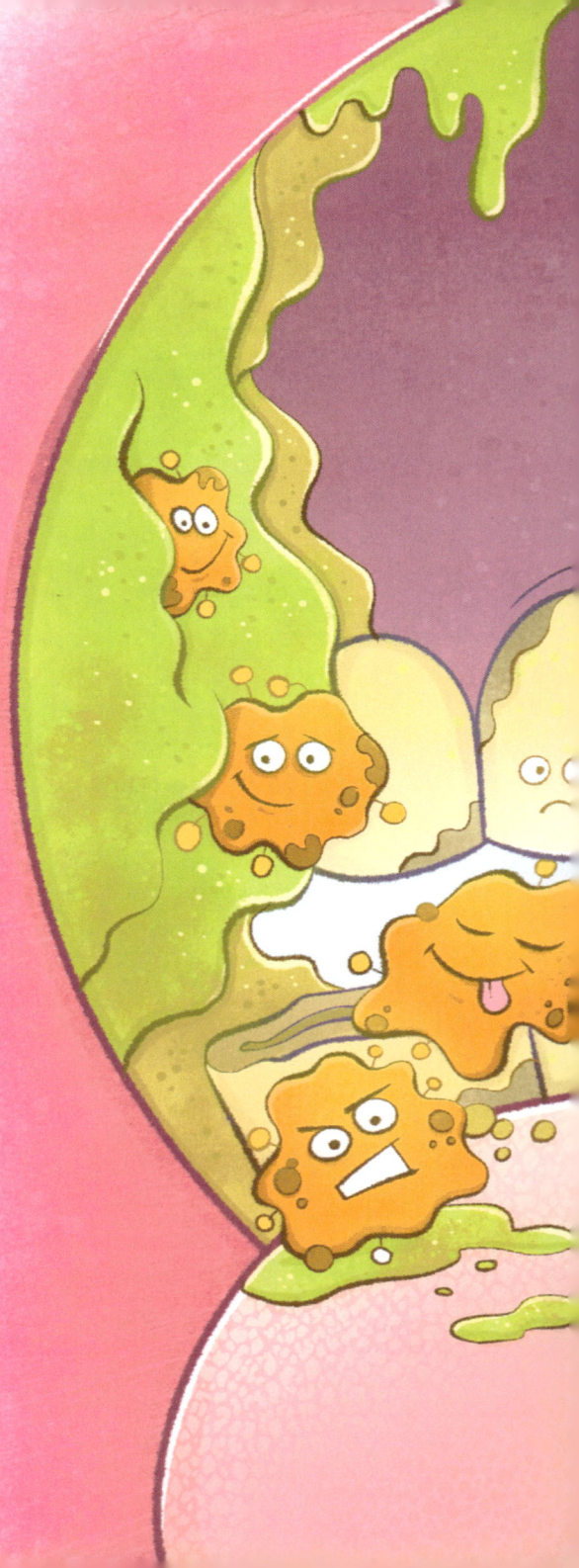

Our teeth become furry, our mouth is so dry,
holes in our teeth and they might make us cry.

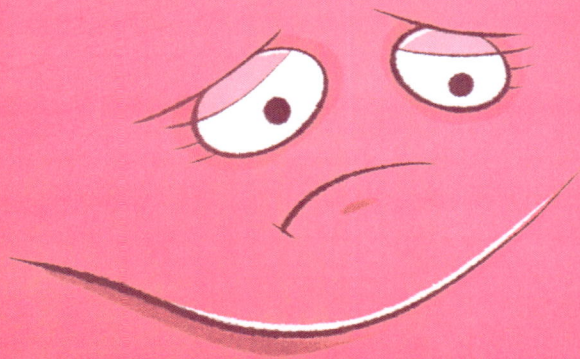

Dear Harry so fun and so helpful before,
Too far from his close friend... so helpful, no more.

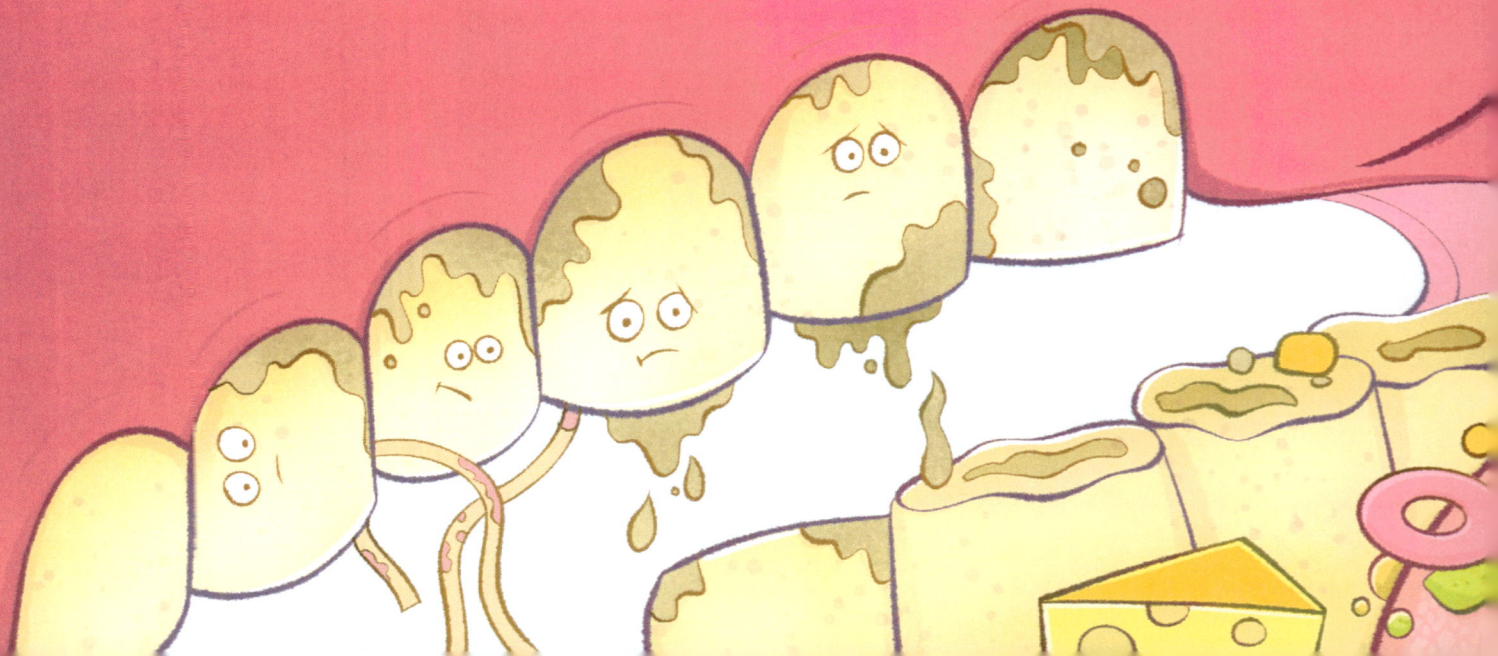

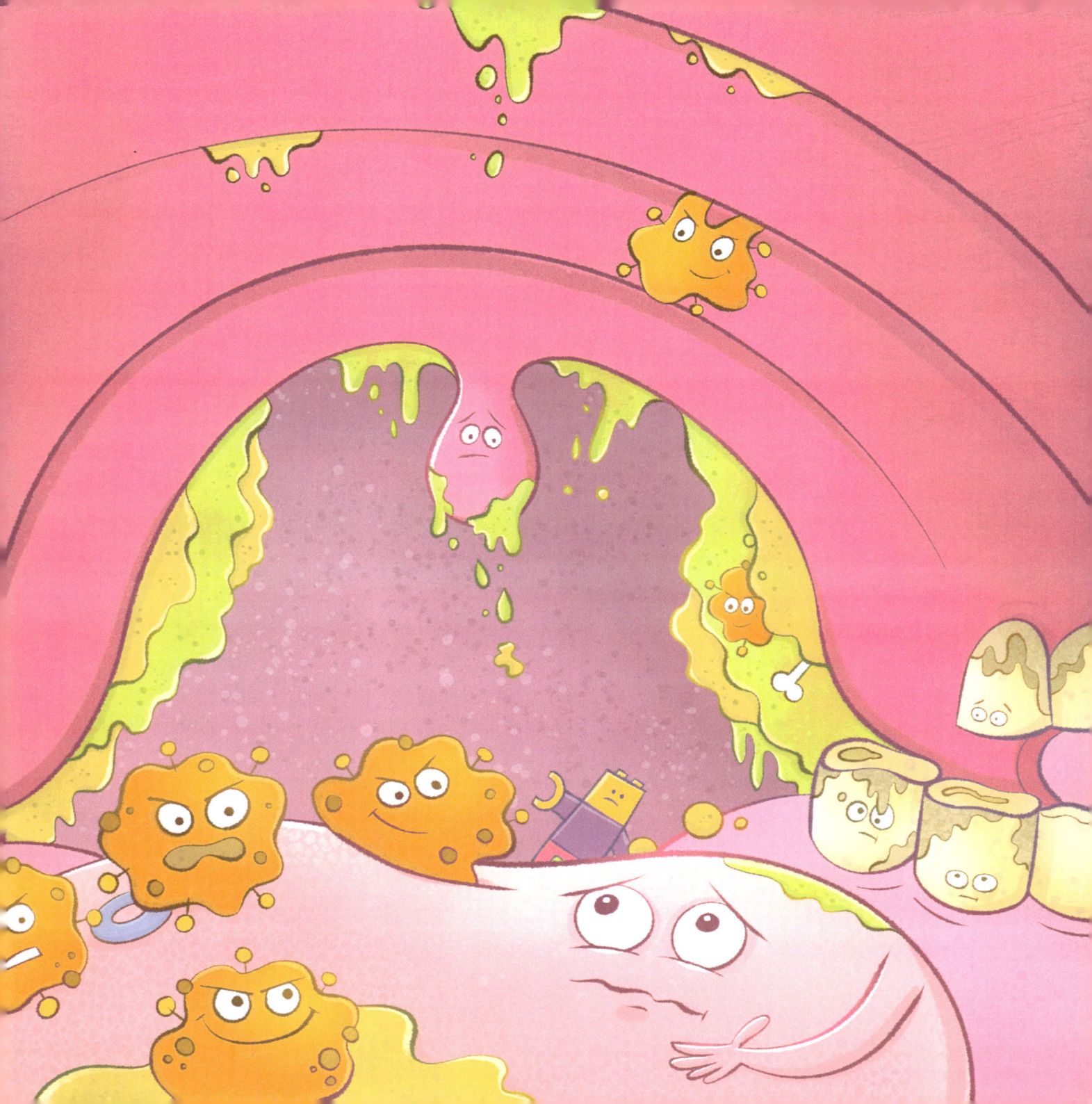

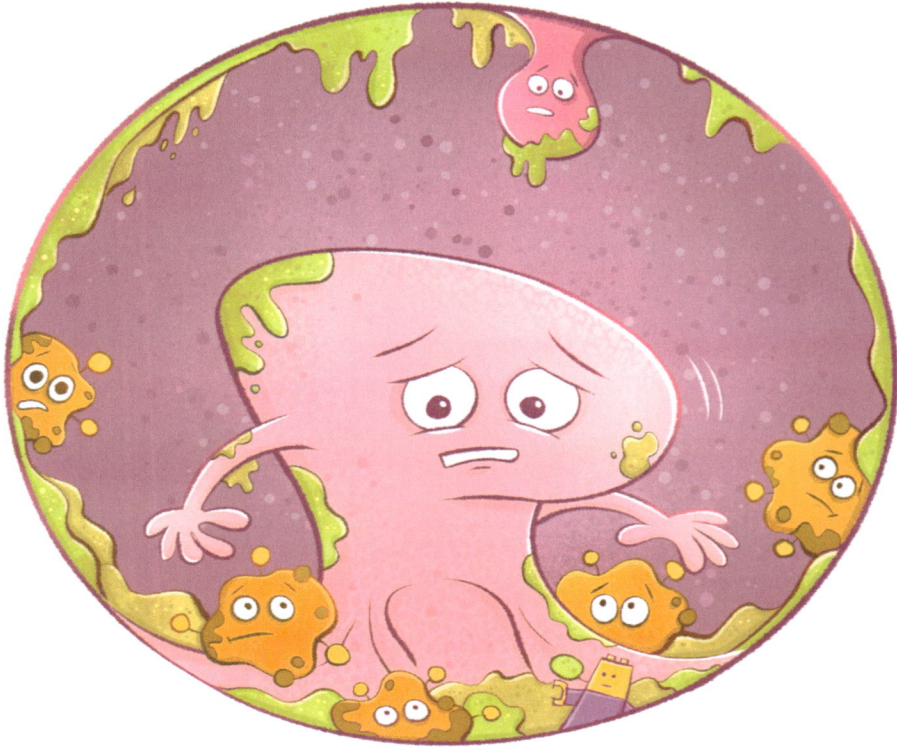

He builds up some courage to stretch his long trunk,
he pushes and wiggles, but feels it has shrunk.

He stretches and reaches to close the big gap,
Closer and closer, gives Polly a tap!

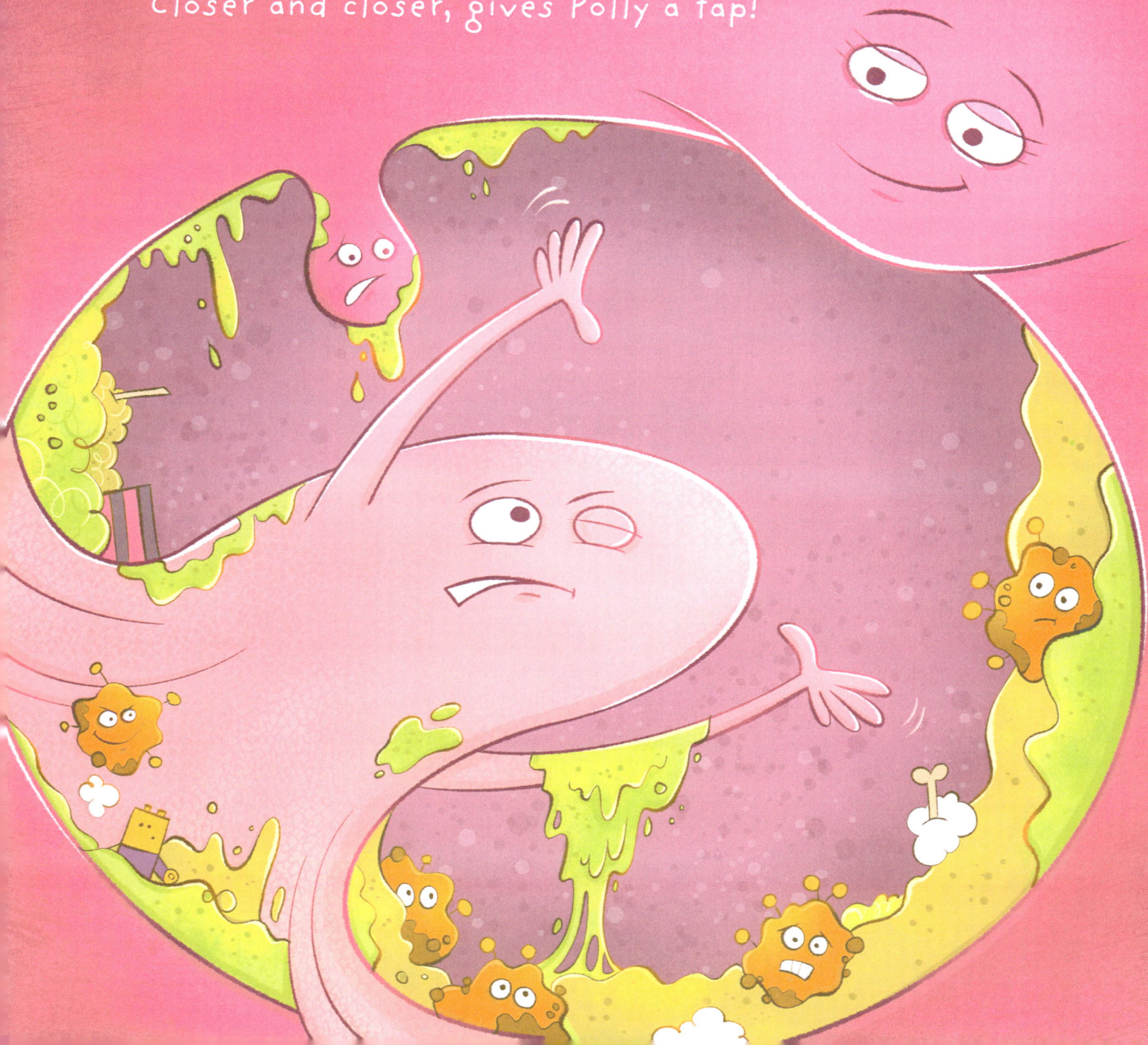

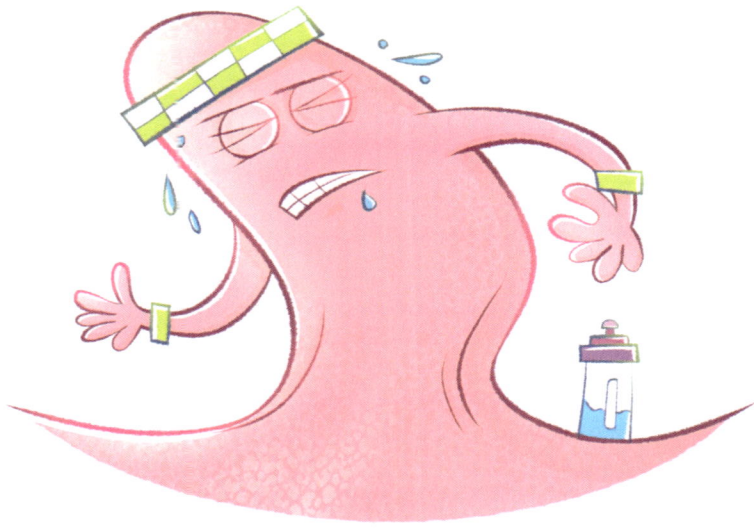

It works! He reaches!
He does it again.

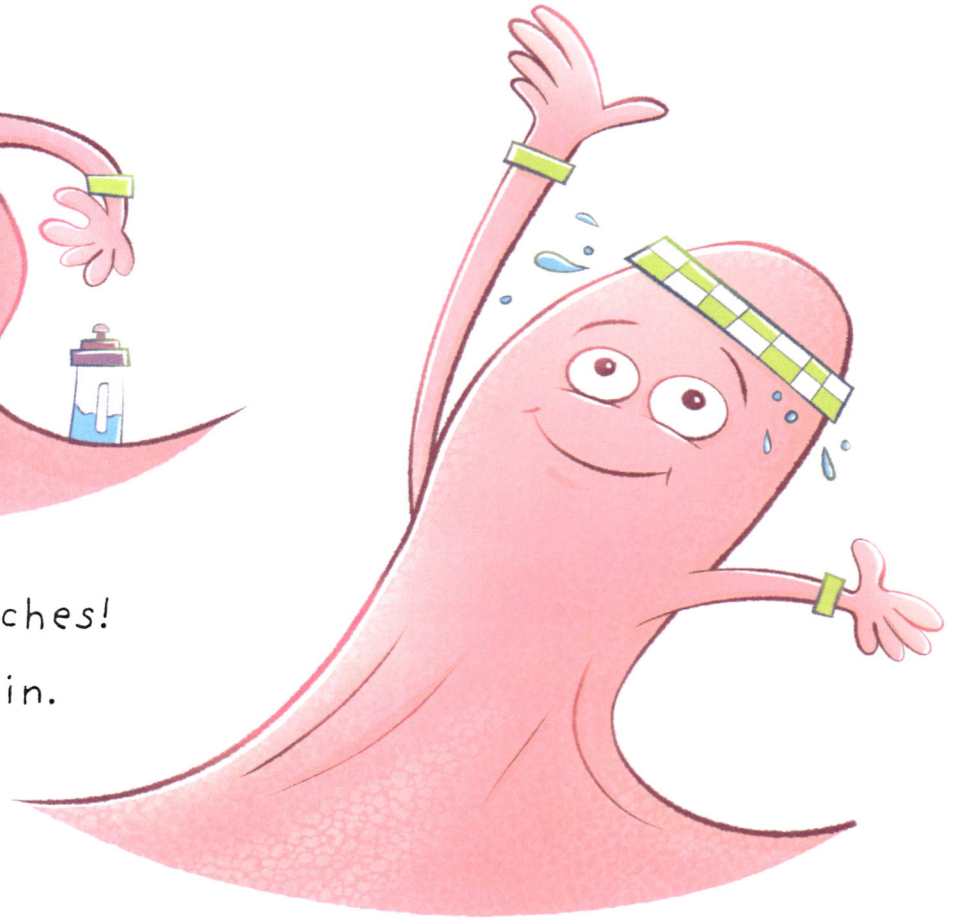

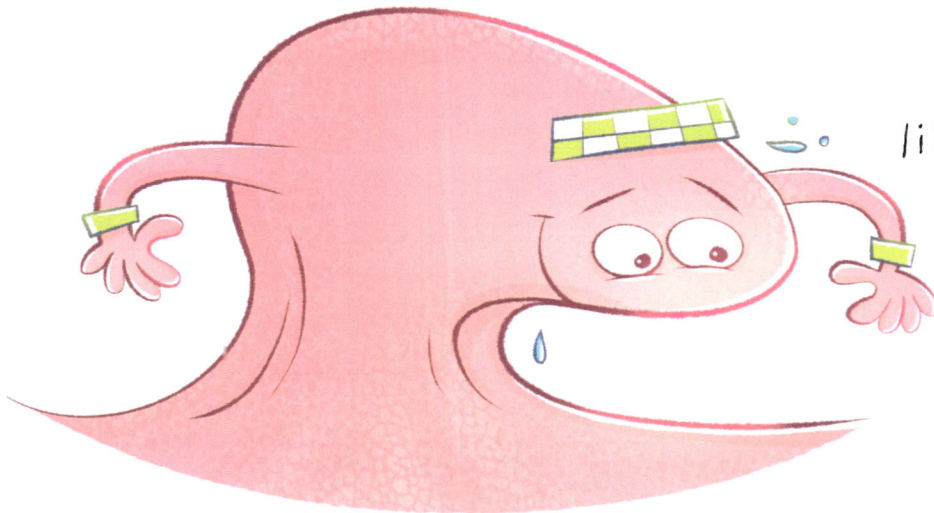

He practices hard
like writing with pen.

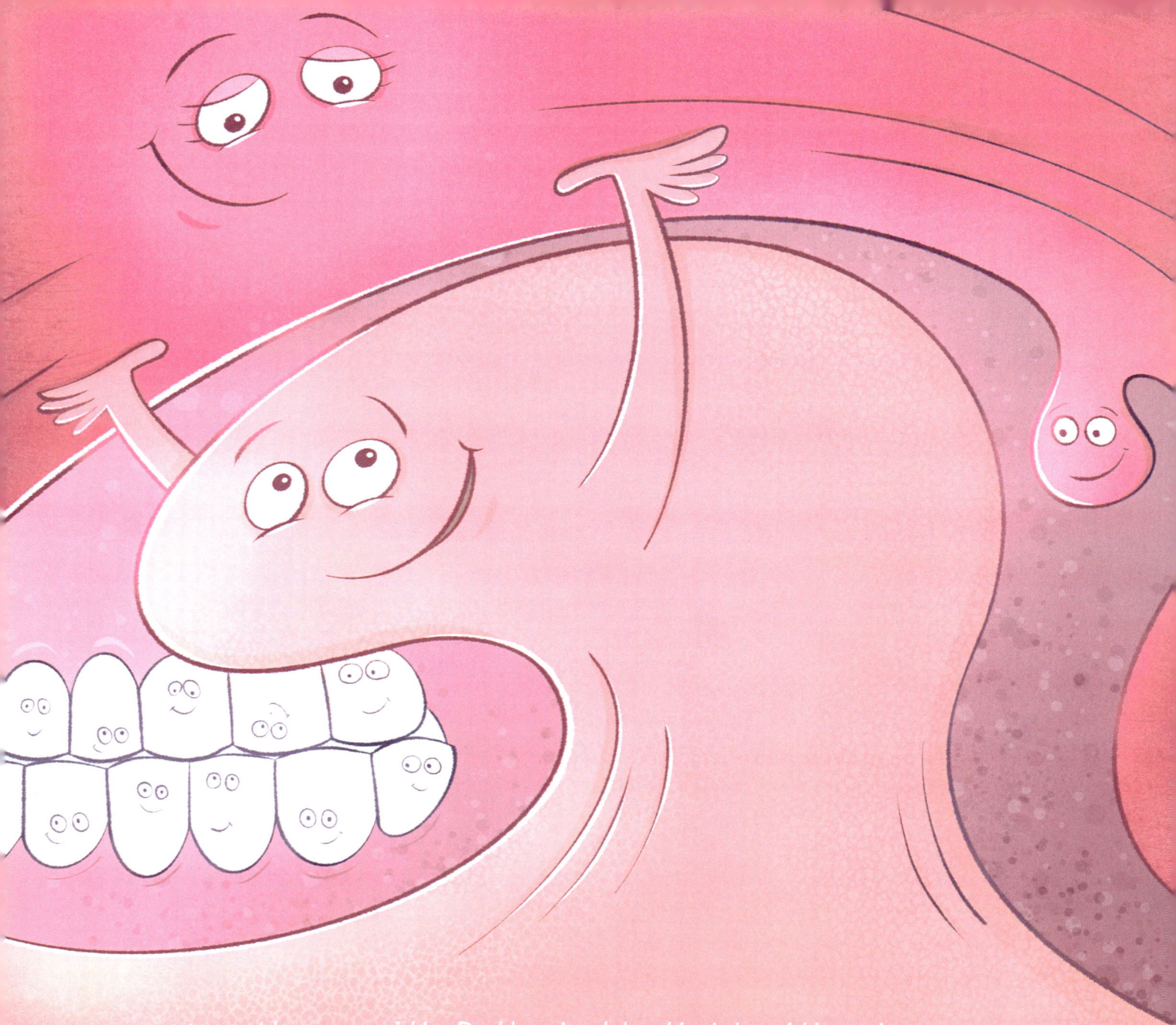

Now Harry with Polly, holds tight with a hug,
Seals off the front door, is snug as a bug.

Our Helpful Harry, now where he should be,
The right place for Harry to live is the key...

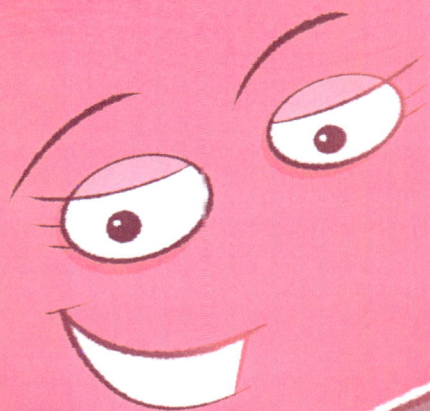

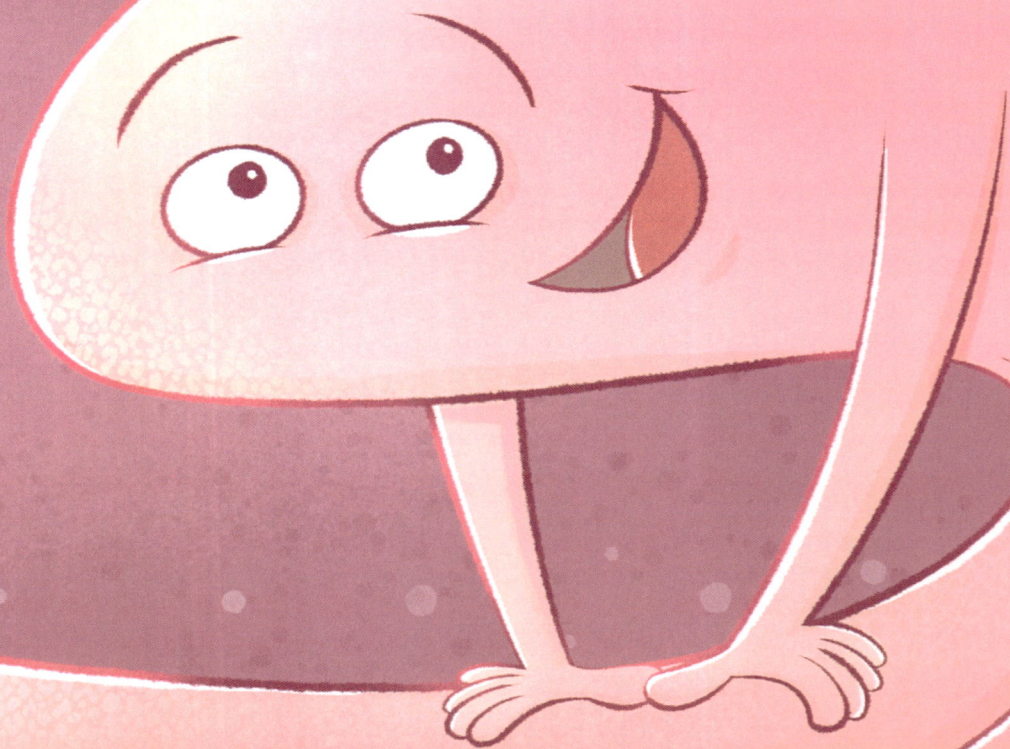

Hugging Miss Polly, best friends, you can see,

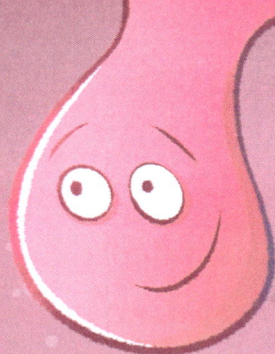

the more that he stretches,
the healthier we'll be!

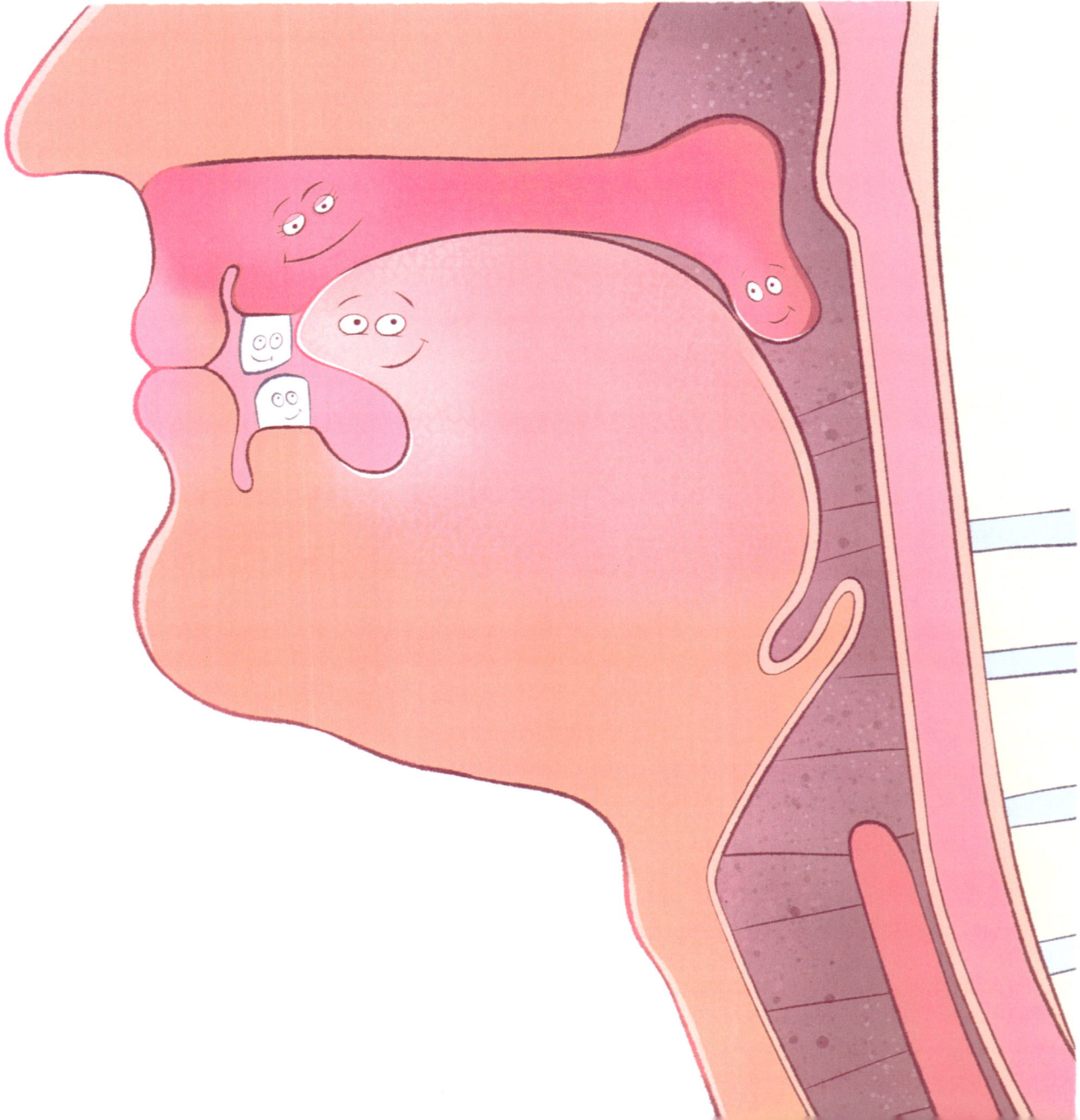

Correct Tongue Postion

Note to parents, caregivers and educators:

Correct tongue posture promotes healthy nasal breathing by sealing off the oral cavity, supporting palatal shape, growth patterns and skeletal structures of the face, settling the central nervous system by stimulating the vagus nerve in the palate, restfull sleep and improved oxygenation to the whole body.

Factors that contribute to the disruption of this posture can include oral habits such as finger and dummy sucking, oral ties (tongue-ties), allergies, chronic inflammation and obstructions to the airways.

Asessments should be conducted with a team of professionals to effectively screen and manage children and adults displaying dysfunctional habits.

Symptoms may include:
- mouth breathing
- snoring/heavy breathing
- clenching/grinding (bruxism)
- persistent thumb, finger and dummy sucking
- crowded teeth
- poor bite
- head, neck and jaw pain
- rampant caries (tooth decay)

Common specialists that can assist in correction may include:
- Airway screening by ENT (Ear Nose and Throat) surgeon
- Allergen testing
- Blood testing
- Dental examinations
- Myofunctional therapy
- Naturopathy, dietetics
- Occupational Therapy
- Osteopathy, chiropractic, massage and physiotherapy
- Orthodontic assessment
- Sleep study
- Speech therapy
- Swallow studies

Simple activities that can be employed to improve muscle tone, coordination, breathing and rest posture to begin the process of improved quality of life and promoting correct growth patterns.

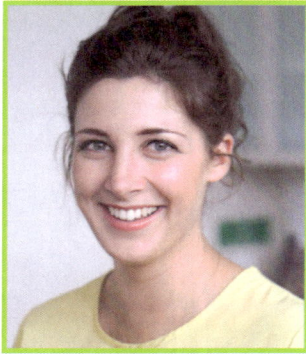

Chantelle Nowicki

Chantelle Nowicki is an Oral Health Therapist and Orofacial Myologist.

She holds "Matter of Face" instagram feed in which she educates viewers about oral health care and function whilst working as a practitioner in private practice since 2010.

"Helpful Harry" being her first piece of written literature, she strives to educate young and old in myofunctional health care in a playful and lighthearted way. She hopes to see vital education delivered in this way to be more receptive to different learning styles and inspire interest in younger generations. Working closely with children specifically in myofunctional therapy, providing a book that covers much of what is taught is a beneficial way of reaching a wider community. She hopes her audience enjoys the fun lighthearted approach to health education that she thrives on.

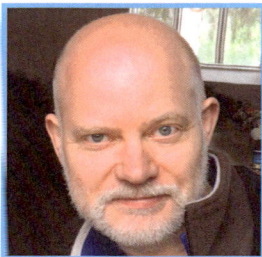

Vaughan Duck

Vaughan loves drawing pictures that make kids giggle. He lives downunder in Australia where it's always sunny.

You can visit Vaughan at vaughanduck.com

www.ingramcontent.com/pod-product-compliance
Lightning Source LLC
Chambersburg PA
CBRC091537260326
41914CB00021B/1641